DIRTY WORLD

Life through Keratoconic Eyes

Jason Cousins

Dirty World: Life through Keratoconic Eyes © 2019 by Jason Cousins.

All Rights Reserved.

No part of this book may be reproduced in any form or by any electronic or mechanical means including information storage and retrieval systems, without permission in writing from the author. The only exception is by a reviewer, who may quote short excerpts in a review.

Cover designed by Jason Cousins

First Printing: February 2019

Gratefully dedicated to Dr Callender and his team of volunteers from the University of Waterloo, Ontario, Canada.

Table of Content

Introduction — 5

Early onset difficulties — 8

Looking through every lens — 16

I saw the light, literally — 30

Uncomfortably grateful — 41

A case of OCD — 55

Looking better — 67

Introduction

We often take our vision for granted. We open our eyes each morning expecting to see the sunlight, our spouses, and our children. We take our phones out the minute they vibrate to read the latest text and with very little effort we pull the keyboard up and respond. We get into our cars and even when the day would have taxed every fibre of our being, we switch the ignition on and make our way home.

For many people, however, seeing to carry out basic tasks such as these require some aid. No, not just your average glasses and certainly not your basic contacts.

For persons living with Keratoconus, a rare degenerative eye condition, seeing requires life-long getting used to gas permeable contact lenses that are as uncomfortable as they sound.

Diagnosing Keratoconus, like with many other rare conditions, often comes at the end of a long winding road, travelled for many years. Allowing the brain to create a norm upon which it functions, as for many years it perceives many things to be as the eyes tell it.

The brain, however, gets a very rude awakening and is left to reprogram itself to a new norm, should the road come to an end and vision is corrected.

Certainly, this was my case.

CHAPTER ONE

Early onset difficulties

I'll be honest, I'm not one to recall every single detail about my childhood. My first birthday party or bike, when I lost my first tooth, what I got for

Christmas each year and all the grand little things we sit and reminisce about from time to time, are all one big blur in my head most times. I do remember having a very difficult time in the fourth grade, however. I was nine then but I'm pretty sure the issue existed in the third grade too. I specifically remember it clearly in the fourth because my teacher, Miss Green, became very frustrated with me, for the reason that I maybe had the worst handwriting of any fourth grader she had ever seen. I couldn't keep my words within the lines. My letters were always lopsided and don't get me started on the fact that I wrote in cursive, or what is more locally called joined-up in my home country, Jamaica. My letters we so joined-up you couldn't make them out. I'm pretty sure I must have told my mom about the issue Miss Green was having. That's right, I said Miss Green, because according to me I was doing my best and I thought I wrote fine. I could read it! Guess me being able to read it wasn't good enough. Miss

Green hated my writing though! I remember on one particular instance she actually called the teacher from the neighboring classroom to take a look at a paper I had brought to her to mark. It caught the attention of the other students in the class and we all know how mean fourth graders can be.

There was an underline issue, however. I was having a genuine medical problem that started to manifest itself and for a while, my parents didn't know. I had keratoconus, a degenerative eye condition in which my cornea loses its elasticity and shape as I grow older. It started losing the smooth round shape of a normal eye and became an irregular cone shape. This is impairing, as the cornea helps to control the amount of light that enters the eye and is no longer able to do this effectively when this happens and requires specially designed contacts to correct.

Over the years I've had to find the most basic ways of explaining Keratoconus to many different people, as most persons have never heard of it. I bet you've never either. I've had to come up with an analogy that I've really mastered telling, because I've always gotten the same follow up questions. "Why can't you just get glasses? Why contacts?" So just in case you've thought the same, here it goes.

Picture having a clear bag all crushed up and trying to shine light through it with a flashlight. The light will have a very hard time going through clearly. But if you stretched the bag and hold the flashlight to it, the light goes through a lot smoother. This is what happens when I put my contacts in, they "stretch" or flatten the cornea so the light goes through better. The reason why glasses could never help is that they sit on your nose, they don't actually touch the eye.

The interesting thing is that my right eye progressed a lot faster than my left. You know how doctors say 20/20 means perfect vision? My eyes right now are 200 in the left and only light sensitive in the right. In other words with my left eye covered, I can't make out that big E on the Snellen chart. Trust me, it's way off from being perfect. Something else really interesting is that my two brothers also have the condition, my parents had perfect vision, but by the time we got into our teens, we had to squint our eyes to read or when driving. Of the three of us, I had it the worst though. I know, it's not fair.

CHAPTER TWO

Looking through every lens

Think about all the things you use your eyes to do, like texting or even reading this book right now. Now squint your eyes almost to a close as you read and stay that way for about 30 seconds. Just do it! Pretty please.

Uncomfortable right? Now imagine having to do that every single time you had to read, watch TV or driving. Don't feel too bad for me though, after a while living with Keratoconus you have to get used to it. Scrap that! It becomes a reflex action to just see in general.

The road to diagnosing my condition was as frustrating as living with it. The condition was not very prevalent in my country, and so I figured that many of the optometrists my parents took me to were just unfamiliar with it. I remember on one particular visit to a clinic called Imperial Optical, the optometrist was initially very hopeful that at the end of the visit he'd be able to find the right lens for me and have me fitted with glasses. I must have sat in that chair for over two hours. I remember us going back and forth trying all types of lenses of various thickness to no avail. I remember as he completed a box he opened another and switching different combinations to find one that could provide my eyes with some semblance of functional vision. It alludes me now but I'm very doubtful we got past the third line on that Snellen chart.

My experience at Imperial Optical was very similar to other experiences I had with other optometrists throughout my middle and high school years. Making an appointment, being hopeful

I'll be fitted with glasses and finally moving on with my life. Only to be disappointed at the end of each visit and not having a word as to what could have been wrong.

My impaired vision affected most aspects of my life, and as you'd imagine, it was very evident in my academics. No, I wasn't a dropout. I wasn't that bad.

You know how they say some people are visual learners? That it's good when we're able to both see and hear during the learning process so our brains can make better connections, so we're better able to memorize what is being thought? Well, if I wanted that, I had to put in some extra effort.

For one I always had to sit at the front of the class, and I was always squinting. I also remember asking my teachers to use darker colored whiteboard makers. Red nor green was no good for me. Black or blue was more my style.

I remember one particular instance very clearly in high school, during a science experiment where we were learning how to use the microscope. I remember the whole class was excited about this experiment because we all had seen microscopes in cartoons like Dexter's Laboratory and Jimmy Neutron our whole lives, but most if not all of us had never seen much more used one in real life. The experiment involved us going outside to pick a tree leaf, treat it with alcohol I believe it was, and creating a slide using a scalpel to remove some of its tissue. The teacher, Mrs. Williams, who I loved very much by the way, then instructed us to view that slide under the microscope at high power and draw two adjacent plant cells. Before we could go ahead with drawing, however, we had to identify these cells with the microscope and have her approve before moving ahead. That's where things got very interesting!

I remember the feeling I had mounting my slide and fastening it to the stage. I remember switching on the light and using the objective lenses, first to scanning then onto low power and finally to high. I was strategic in my search, looking through the eyepiece and viewing one end of my specimen to another to find the perfect two cells to draw. I remember her saying we should search for cells that we could distinguish as much cell organelles in as possible. So I made sure I was very selective in my choice. Finally, I decided on my two lucky cells. I remember I could have clearly identified the nucleus and cell wall as well as what I thought were mitochondria. So as she instructed, I called her to view my cell choices.

Now I remember I had to wait a bit to have her come over to me because she was seeing another student, but throughout the wait time I was very sure that nothing disturbed my microscope. So I was very surprised about what happened next.

She came over and started viewing my slide through the eyepiece and asked me "what am I looking at?" I was a little bit surprised by the question but still, with enthusiasm, I answered, "my two cells." Then she said something to the effect "no, you need to focus your microscope properly" and walked off to another student.

Now I was a little perturbed because from what I saw I thought my two cells were perfect for the exercise. I remember when she walked off I looked at my microscope just to see if it was actually set to high power because I was a little confused as to what had just happened. It was, but who was I to argue with Mrs. Williams. She was awesome.

Starting from the top like a good student, I removed my slide, remounted it and started searching again for cells. They really weren't hard to find this time around since I knew their general location. Again like she instructed us, I asked her to come and see, and again she did. To my disappointing surprise again she said my microscope was very much unfocused and she wasn't seeing anything, which I found very strange because I was seeing my cells very clearly. She then attempted to assist me by focusing the eyepiece to clearly see the cells. What was really interesting was that when she focused it and I looked, I couldn't make out one thing!

Much like when I focused it and she looked.

Eventually, she figured out what was happening and told me that I was using the microscope to compensate for my vision impairment and so someone with a more "normal" vision would not be able to see it clearly if I were to focus it. Would you imagine that?!

CHAPTER THREE

I saw the light, literally

When I think of it sometimes, it's quite a difficult position to be in, being ill most of your life in some way or another and not knowing what really is wrong. Visiting different doctors and each time hoping for at least a name. Something to start researching or even pray about. Something to tell someone that asks why I had to squint so much. For me, I didn't get a name until 2003, when I was 16 years old.

That year, my mom got word of a public clinic in our country that hosted a team of volunteer optometrists each year from the University of Waterloo in Ontario, Canada. The Foundation for International Self Help Development

(F.I.S.H) clinic located in Kingston, Jamaica. That year, they hosted the expertise I needed to give me the name and diagnoses that so long alluded me. I remember the visit went much like many others before, a general assessment of my vision and then a fitting for the right lens. Like others, the team went through many different lenses trying to find the right one. I think by this time I wasn't even annoyed by it anymore. I just read the chart whenever they said to, being as corporative as possible. But at 16 it was hard to not become irritated and not feel as if this was not as hopeless as other times before it. I was to be pleasantly surprised, however.

I remember we were in a very small room and the optometrists talked together for a while and then told me they were going to "try something". Of course, trusting in them completely, I was up for anything they had in mind. After all, we had gotten nowhere with anyone nor anything else before. I wasn't expecting what they proposed next though.

They got a single contact lens and said they were going to fit me with it. Now initially, I was a little bit anxious about that. To this point, I had never had anything larger than a speck of dust or an eyelash in my eye, and even then it was the most annoying thing ever and like anyone else I'd just want it out. So the thought of having a piece of plastic in my eye was something to get used to. But, I was willing to give it a shot, and

I did, and what happened next was nothing short of life changing.

You see, up to that point I was never able to see details or literally the "finer things in life." I was never able to make out wrinkles or pimples on my face or on anyone else's. I was never able to make out trees or houses along a hillside, all I could ever make out were green patches interspersed with roadways. I was never able to make out birds flying or perched in a tree, nor truly enjoy an eclipse, a rainbow nor a starry night's sky. I'd hear airplanes flying over our community and couldn't actually see them. That was all about to change, however, and I couldn't wait!

It took a while before they could get the contact into my eye, I can't recall if it was the left or the right, but I recall closing it every time they attempted to place it in. I wasn't being difficult or anything, honestly, it was just by reflex. If you've ever worn contacts then you've certainly experienced that awkward first time putting it in. The eye is just not used to anything touching it like that so the eyelids would put up a fight and keep closing.

They eventually gave in and we were able to get the contact in, but the next battle was to get it in the right position over the pupil. It kept shifting all over my eye, from one end to another. The feeling was horrible! But I fought through it and we eventually got it right. Now I know your next question might be, "did it work, did someone light a match at the end of the dark, long keratoconic tunnel?" And the answer is, YES!

I think when we got the lens in I started blinking about one thousand times per minute, but for every millisecond they were opened, I could see! My eyes were running like a small river, but what the heck, I could see! The whole time I felt like I wanted to pluck the eye out, but again, I could see! I remember the first thing I looked at was my forearm, I remember I started laughing because I never knew my arm was so hairy! My next sight is one to remain in my memory forever though. I turned and I looked at my mom, and I saw her in all her beauty. I finally saw why many people said I resembled her.

After a little while to soak it all in, the doctors and I got back to business. They asked me to close the other eye and read the Snellen chart another time. I can't quite remember how far down I was able to get this time around, but I'm pretty sure it was further than I've ever gotten before. It was enough for the doctors to finally give us a diagnosis, Keratoconus.

They then explained to my mom and me what it was and why it was so difficult to diagnose. At first, it was much like Spanish to us but like any tech-savvy teen would do, I got home and googled it and I read as much as I could find. After all, how could I not, I now had a name.

CHAPTER FOUR

Uncomfortably grateful

Finally having a diagnosis meant more to me than I could ever express. It meant getting the answer to a lifelong question, and that's priceless. Or so I thought. Finally having a diagnosis also meant finally getting it corrected, and we quickly learned how costly the condition would be. After my visit to the FISH clinic, where I was seen by the greatest set of volunteer optometrists in the history of volunteering optometrists, I was referred to a local doctor who would help me to manage the condition from then on. So on August 14th, 2003, I had my first visit with Dr. Woo-Lawson of the Optical Zone.

I remember much of the details of my first conversation with Dr. Woo-Lawson. For one, for the whole visit I kept thinking to myself, why didn't we discover this place before? It would have saved us so much trouble, headache, and money. I recall asking her why so many doctors could not have diagnosed the condition and she confirmed my previous thought that it was just not very prevalent and well known locally. She told me what the prospects were for living with Keratoconus and that I'd be considered legally blind by the age of 30 if it continued to progress the way it was. She told me what the corrective measures were, and that ultimately I would require a corneal transplant. Yes, that's exactly what it sounds like. I'd get a dead man's cornea. Of course, you know that didn't sit very well with me. She, however, said that this was the last resort because of how risky the procedure is. But until then, I'd be wearing contacts.

The assessment began pretty normally, going through the routine to ascertain the state of my vision. This time things felt a bit different, however. This time, knowing exactly what was wrong and what would be needed to correct it, made me lose the hopefulness I had with every change of lens, as with the previous examinations. Hopeful that the next would maybe be the right one. But it did feel amazing to know this time around our efforts, time and money were no longer being wasted. Knowing exactly what we were up against.

Eventually, the assessment process went from switching glasses lenses to switching contact lenses. Now, upon till then, I had only worn a single contact once and only for a brief period, during my visit to the FISH clinic. And that was one single lens. This time around I was being fitted for both eyes and I had never felt anything like it before.

She started with the right eye, it is the worse and the one in which the condition had developed the furthest. The difficulty with fitting contacts for a condition like a keratoconus is finding one that would correct the vision yet offer as much comfort considering the ill shape of the eye's cornea and that these lenses were not the normal soft lenses. The lenses used in correcting Keratoconus are called gas permeable lenses, and they are very hard!

It took a great deal of time and patience, but like the trooper I am, I pulled through and we eventually found the best fit for each eye. Each lens at the time cost about $300 US dollars and we made the payment for both. The doctor told us that they were not made locally but she would have to have them made and shipped by an overseas company, and that it would take approximately twenty business days. Twenty long, anxiety-filled, couldn't wait until they were over business day. It ultimately took a bit longer but I had no complaints, I had waited 16 years for that day and to wait for a few more was a breeze. A mixed emotions breeze, but a breeze nonetheless.

They finally arrived and the receptionist called my mom to say we wouldn't need to schedule another appointment, I could just come in at any time for a brief session. I got there the next day, all by myself this time, and we started by immediately fitting my eyes with the new lenses and an assessment using the Snellen chart. Dr. Woo-Lawson told me the lenses improved my vision to 20/20 and I believed her, I could read every line of the chart! We then went over to another room and then things started getting interesting, at least in my head.

Up until that point, the doctor was always the one to fit the contacts in my eye and the normally she would immediately turn the lights off in the room. And this along with the fact that my blinking rate quadrupled every time I had it in, prevented me from ever taking in the sight of anything around me. But this time, in this well-lit room, I got a chance to, and as I looked around and even on myself, I couldn't help starting to feel unfamiliar.

I saw details I had never perceived before in my life. I saw marks on my skin I never knew were there and again I saw how hairy it was. I took a look in a mirror that was before me and saw that I had truly inherited early greying from my dad and grandfather as one side of my hair was almost covered in white. My nails were not as clean as I had thought they were and my teeth weren't as white. I started thinking that nothing was really how I perceived them and what scared me the most was that this was just by myself in one small room. I had a world to go face very shortly.

Dr. Woo-Lawson started to give me a rundown of how to care for my lenses and said it was my time to practice putting them in and removing them. While she spoke with me, I couldn't help noticing all the details on her face.

Things I had never seen before, wrinkles, pimples, and make-up. Don't get me wrong, she was beautiful, just that I was only then taking note of these things.

At the end of the session, I was torn between wearing them home and taking them out and waiting until I got home to refit them. Though by then I knew I was in for a few visual surprises along the way, I couldn't help being excited about just being able to see clearly. So I decided to take them for a spin.

CHAPTER FIVE

A case of OCD

I think I can explain my very first response to facing sunlight using this analogy I'm pretty sure you're familiar. You know how vampires respond to the sunlight in those scary movies when their pray somehow survives until sunrise and kicks a window? And in pure anguish, the vampire flees to the darkest part of the room he could find? That was my exact response!

I felt like my eyes were going to catch fire. I had to seek shade and close my eyes every chance I got, my whole journey home. Whenever I was able to, however, I didn't fail to take in as much as I could. And in my head at least, it was the small room experience all over again. In short, nothing was as clean as I thought they were. Ironically, now with brighter, clearer vision, everything seemed a lot dirtier! And it felt weird. I felt anxious. That same feeling of unfamiliarity crept over me.

I remember looking at the cars as they passed and knowing from then on that people don't actually wash their cars as often as I thought. And I questioned why I thought sidewalks were cleaner than they actually were. I remember standing at the bus park, about to take public transport for the first time with my new contacts. I would read everything in sight, literally. I would read some things twice just because I now could. I was finally able to read bus numbers from afar off. And I recalled many times buses would have passed me by because I was too late at fanning them down, simply because they'd have to be very near for me to make out the number. But not that day.

As with most of the vehicles, I saw that day, the bus was dirty. I could see where someone, a child may be, had written in the dirt presumably with their fingers. I remember feeling like an alien stepping on the mothership for the first time in a long time. Looking at everything with discerning eyes. There was graffiti, some garbage and of course, dirt. The seats were either stained, torn or both.

The journey home felt much like a tour. Though without an actual guide, the excitement and anticipation I felt about seeing with my new vision, some of the usual sights on my way home, was enough to keep me pumped. The billboards, the buildings, and malls were some of the few things running through my head. I also thought about my street. What would it look like? What about my house? I was especially dying to see my room and my family.

Where I lived in Kingston was a mountainous area. In a valley actually. But I was never able to fully appreciate its beauty, until that day. They were the first things to catch my eyes as I came off the bus. They were green! No, not just one big green cloud like I used to perceive, but I could actually make out trees. Even to the peak. I could make out actual houses and roads leading up.

If any of my neighbors saw me walking down my road that day they would have thought I was being weird. I remember looking at every house as if it were the first time seeing them. The street like most I had seen up until then was dirty. Not horribly dirty. But as dirty as the streets get. It was normal. Just for me, a new more detailed vision came with a new normal. One I had to get use to.

My dogs would always greet me on the way in, and I usually just casually patted them on the head and asked if they missed me. That day I took a little more time to greet them, however. I had two ridgebacks, Black Rhino, and his mom Kartel. Black Rhino was of course, black, with a really shiny coat he had gotten from his dad. A lot shinier than I had previously thought now that I had HD vision. His mom Kartel was of a light brown color.

My mom was the only one home that day. And she was as excited about my new vision as I was. She had been on this journey with me the whole time and she was anxious to know how I was finding them. I had mixed emotions heading into the house, however. Mixed because they were flat out uncomfortable, but yet provided me with the vision I could have only dreamed of before. When I got into the house she had a huge smile on her face. She was watching TV but flew up from the chair to ask me the inevitable question. "How are they?" Again I saw in detail how beautiful my mom was and I told her exactly how I felt the whole way home. Excellent vision but at an uncomfortable price.

She was quick to notice a major change that had taken place. I was looking at the TV but I was not squinting. I was actually reading the TV guide from the furthest couch in the living room. This made her smile more.

I remember looking around in the living room and the paint on the walls much like Black Rhino's coat was a lot richer in color. I made my way to the other parts of the house looking around as if I was on a real estate tour. There was one familiar thread running through my day's experience and as I feared, it made its ways straight to my bedroom. Dirt! My walls were in dire need of painting! There were dirt stains everywhere. What I thought was a white painted room was actually mostly brown with white anywhere hands and feet couldn't reach. There was one particular dirt mark on the wall at the end of my bed. I knew it was there, as I had a habit of putting my feet up whenever I would use my phone on my bed. But man, I never knew it was that ugly!

CHAPTER SIX

Looking better

Most everyone I knew and interacted with regularly quickly noticed a difference in how I was seeing. Which for me spoke to how obviously bad it was before contacts. I remember many of my friends saying they noticed I wasn't squinting anymore, and I no longer had to hold things two inches from my face to read. Sometimes I'd allow them to pick these things up before I told them what had happened. Or depending on who it was, I'd become so excited to see them with my new vision that they'd think I was being weird and I'd just have to tell them.

After leaving high school at seventeen, I worked for a while in a local pharmaceutical company until I was nineteen years old. After which I attended community college pursuing advance biology and chemistry, and worked on getting into medical school. Things didn't work out quite as I planned for financial reasons, but life was a lot better being able to see clearly. Though I didn't get to complete med school, I couldn't have imagined doing a course such as anatomy without my contacts. Or trying to keep up in a two-hour lecture having to squint at every slide.

Throughout my life, I've always had mixed emotions about my vision. Wait, let me explain. So like any impairment, of course, it's annoying and I wish things were otherwise. Of course, I would have loved to have a 20/20 vision my whole life. Who wouldn't?! But for some strange, parallel universe reason, however, I don't believe I wouldn't have reservations if I could start things over differently. Again, let me explain. My vision has been a topic of conversation, an ice breaker and a binding agent for many relationships

I've had throughout my life. It has given me, my family and friends so many experiences of laughter that I couldn't imagine life without many of them sometimes. So, yes, it's been a rough road, but one with many points I'm thankful for.

www.ingramcontent.com/pod-product-compliance
Lightning Source LLC
Chambersburg PA
CBHW021505210526
45463CB00002B/900